Beverly Physical Therapist

Discovers the **Truth** about Plantar Fasciitis

by Chris Dukarski, PT

DISCLAIMER:

The information provided in this book is designed to provide helpful information
on the subjects discussed. This book is not meant to be used, nor should it be
used, to diagnose or treat any medical condition. For diagnosis or treatment of
any medical problem, consult your own physician.

The publisher and author are not responsible for any specific medical
or health needs that may require supervision by a licensed healthcare
practitioner, and thus they are not liable for any consequences from any
recommendation, to any person reading or following the information in
this book.

OUCH!! MY FOOT HURTS!!

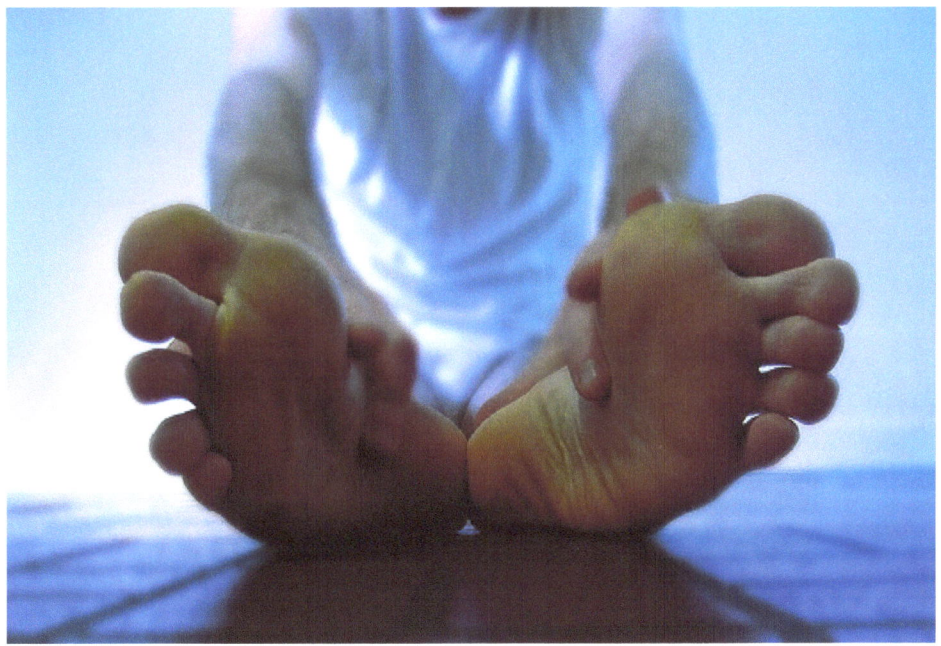

There are a lot of people out there suffering from foot pain. Whether it be plantar fasciitis, pain in the ball of the foot or simply "pain in the foot"!! They turn to the internet or You Tube looking for answers.

Looking for the cure-all.
Looking for the quick fix.

But I have to tell you…it isn't there. There is no quick fix for most people. Sure, you hear stories about the miracle manipulation or acupuncture session or cortisone shot. But I've got to tell you, for most people, it isn't there. So, what do you do; you keep on searching.

Looking
Hoping.
Until one day you hit the breaking point.

So what do most people do NEXT
You call your doctor or you get referred to a therapist.
All doctors and therapists are created equal - right?
WRONG!
Maybe you get partial relief after 6 weeks of
therapy or after a cortisone shot.
6 weeks of copays
Deductible?
Did you have to pay out-of-pocket?

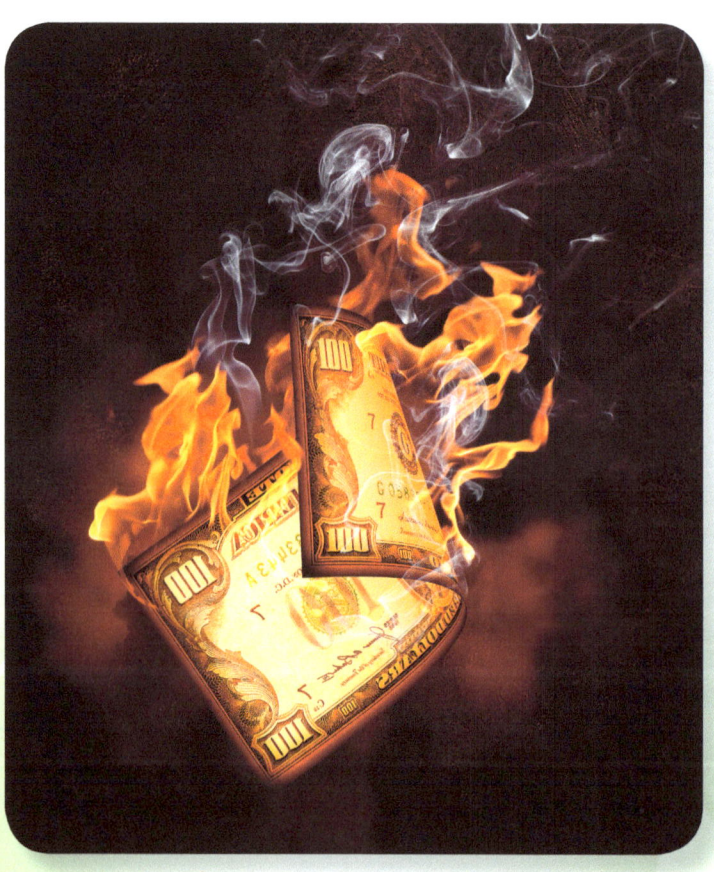

Now you may be right back to square one.
Just a little poorer
And maybe a little angrier…

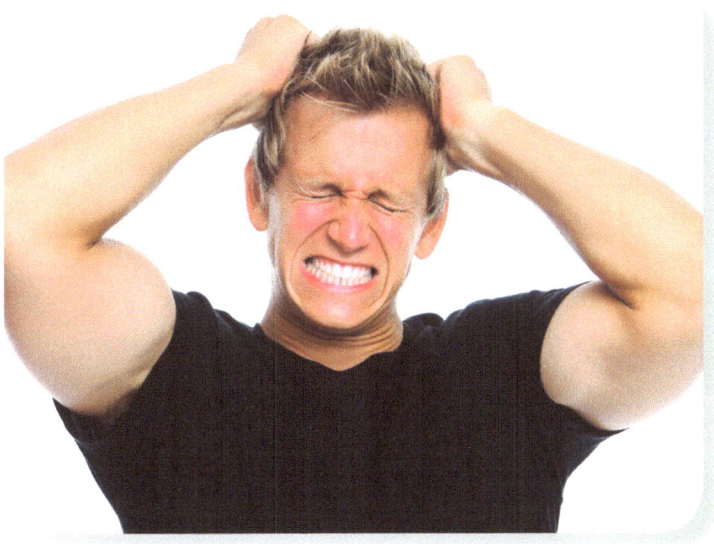

I can't tell you how many times in my 22 years as a Physical Therapist that I have heard similar stories. I have heard and felt the frustration and anger. I have empathized with my patients who have suffered longer than they should have to because our system is a "little" broken. HMO's are restricting your access. Health care systems are tightening their belts under the guise of "Accountable Care Organizations" or ACO's. Your deductibles and copays are getting higher. It is this energy combined with my own passion and tenacity that encouraged me to open my specialty physical therapy clinic. I knew that there was a better way to provide effective, comprehensive and evidenced based physical therapy. My patients are my best advocates.

"I had been to two PT's with little success..Chris and his staff are part of a cutting-edge, welcoming, and success-oriented program that I'd recommend to anyone."- J.W.

"I play for a division one sports team at the University of Pennsylvania. I have gone to see many specialists looking for solutions and had not found the answer until coming to WalkWell."- M.W.

"I had gone to PT for 3 months before coming to WalkWell. I am now painfree. "-M.V.

"After 6 years of pain, I have my life back. Chris never gave up on me!!" -M.B.

"After OrthoWell, my second marathon time was better that my first... when I was 10 years younger." -C.H.

"The individual attention and rehab is without peer. And on the 8th day, God created WalkWell." -T.L.

I want to share with you what I've learned and refined over 22 years of thoughtful and engaging physical therapy.

There's a very good reason for all that I do. I have seen the videos. I have followed the blogs. I have analyzed peer-reviewed research. I have done the work for you.

My techniques…
My protocols…
My approach to YOUR health…
WORKS

KNOWLEDGE IS POWER!!

I'm sure that you will agree that there is a LOT of information on-line about foot pain and plantar fasciitis. My intention with this book is to open your eyes to some things that you may NOT have read. I want you to understand what the experts have discovered. I want to open the door of controversy over the role that inflammation, cortisone shots, and foot orthotics may or may not be playing in terms of your pain.

You need to UNDERSTAND your foot pain. You need to understand the most common "pain in the foot" condition – plantar fasciitis!! One United States study estimated that one million patient visits each year are for the diagnosis and treatment of heel pain.[1,7] Plantar fasciitis appears in the sedentary and geriatric population[2,3,4,7], it makes up one quarter of all foot injuries in runners[5,7], and is the reason for 8% of all injuries to people participating in sports.[6,7] I performed a comprehensive literature review on heel pain in order to educate myself and YOU on what the research says regarding the origins of heel pain as well as the research behind physical therapy interventions. So here it is! Knowledge is power! Read on!

WE CANNOT SOLVE OUR PROBLEMS WITH THE SAME THINKING WE USED WHEN WE CREATED THEM
- Albert Einstein

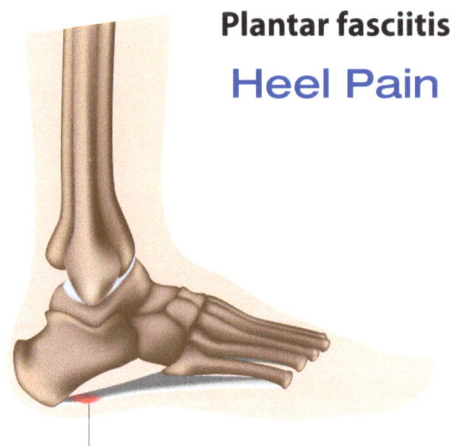

Plantar fasciitis

Heel Pain

Inflammation of the plantar fascia

THE EVIDENCE

Heel pain is a very common and painful condition. One United States study estimates that one million patient visits each year are for the diagnosis and treatment of plantar heel pain.[1,7] This disorder appears in the sedentary and geriatric population[2,3,4,7], it makes up one quarter of all foot injuries in runners[5,7], and is the reason for 8% of all injuries to people participating in sports.[6,7] The exact nature of the disorder as well as the most appropriate treatment, however, remains unclear.[7-14] A study of 364 painful heels could find no causal relationship.[15] Few random, controlled studies document the efficacy of conservative care,[7,10,13,17,18] yet success rates for conservative treatment of plantar heel pain vary from 46% to 100% in the literature.[8,9,14] It becomes clear from a review of the literature that the etiology of plantar heel pain is multi-factorial i.e. "multiple etiology heel pain syndrome." There is not one specific cause, nor is there a panacea for conservative treatment. In 1972, Snook and Chrisman[16] wrote" it is reasonably certain that a condition which has so many different theories of etiology and treatment does not have valid proof of any one cause". Are we any better off today?

The management of plantar heel pain begins with the correct differential diagnosis.[11,19,20] Plantar fasciitis is the most common diagnosis for plantar heel pain.[21] Clinical findings include medial heel pain which is often worse in the morning, worse after periods of rest, worse after prolonged weight bearing activity, and pain to palpation at the medial/plantar heel.[11,22] Most researchers agree that the pain is caused by microtrauma to the origin of the plantar fascia at the medial tubercle of the calcaneus.[22-25] Subsequently, this microtrauma causes marked thickening and fibrosis at the origin of the plantar fascia. Many practitioners believe that the pain of plantar fasciitis is caused by inflammation.[18,27-30] However, researchers have shown through histological examination that there is an absence of inflammatory cells in chronic overuse tendinopathies.[29-36] Animal studies conclusively demonstrate that, within 2-3 wks of insult to tendon tissue, inflammatory cells are not present.[31-35] Histologic findings from plantar fasciotomies have been presented to support the thesis that plantar fasciitis is a degenerative fasciosis without inflammation, not a fasciitis.[26,31] In addition to the absence of inflammatory cells, tendinosis is characterized by a degeneration of tenocytes and collagen fibers with a subsequent increase in non-collagenous matrix.[31-35] The collagen tissue of tendons, for example, have only 13% of the oxygen uptake of muscle and require >100 days to synthesize collagen.[31-35] Thus, tissue repair in tendinosis may take 3 to 6 months.[31-35] With this increasing body of evidence suggesting fasciosis, not fasciitis, the practitioner needs to shift his/her treatment perspective.

As payers demand practitioners to maximize outcomes and minimize costs, the need for evidence-based interventions becomes clear. As stated above, however, there are few studies that have tested the efficacy of treatment protocols.[7-14,31-35] The first treatment goal for plantar fasciosis should be to protect the healing tissue.[31-35,37-40] How can damaged tissue heal if environmental stresses are not controlled?[38] The second goal should be to restore the normal mechanical behavior of the tissue and to positively influence the structural reorientation of damaged collagen fibers. Physical therapists have proposed that the treatment of plantar heel pain should be impairment based.[41] A detailed examination would identify these impairments and an appropriate plan of care would utilize manual therapy, exercise, and modalitites.[41] There is no standard physical therapy protocol for plantar fasciosis, however, upon review of the literature by this author, a framework of evidence is available to establish an appropriate protocol.

Iontophoresis and corticosteroid injections have been used to treat the proposed presence of inflammation at the origin of the plantar fascia. Iontophoresis is a process that uses bipolar electric fields to propel molecules of a drug such as dexamethasone across intact skin and into underlying tissue.[42] The depth of drug penetration averages 8-12 mm with deeper penetration occurring through a slower process of passive diffusion.[42-44] Two articles have documented an improvement of plantar heel pain using iontophoresis with dexamethasone, yet long term relief was questionable.[45] Steroids have been shown to inhibit the early stages as well as the later manifestations of the inflammatory process.[46] Corticosteroid injections for relief of plantar heel pain have had mixed results.[9-10,11-13,47] However, ultrasound guided peritendinous injections of achilles and patella tendonitis have shown a significant reduction in the average diameter of the affected tendons[46] as well as a disappearance of neovascularization.[48] Improper injection technique may be the reason for unfavorable results.[8]

Tissue protection can occur through rest, activity modification, taping techniques, and foot orthoses. Low-dye taping and various plantar strapping techniques have been shown to be effective in relieving plantar heel pain as well as altering foot kinematics and plantar pressures.[49-54] Although limited evidence exists,[14,55-62] no conclusive evidence has been found to demonstrate the effectiveness of foot orthoses on plantar heel pain.[11-14,55,59]

Manual therapy procedures used by medical practitioners can include soft tissue mobilization, massage, manual traction, joint mobilization, and joint manipulation.[63] Clinical interventions involving joint mobilizations and manipulations have been developed or refined by many authors.[63-68] Although there is clear evidence to justify the use of manual therapy on spinal disorders, there is an absence of controlled trials in peripheral joints.[63] We can only speculate that a relationship exists between the identified joint impairment and the patient's plantar heel pain.[41] There is, however, a body of work that attempts to demonstrate the effect of mobilizations and/or manipulations of the talus and fibula on ankle dorsiflexion range of motion, yet with varied results.[69-73]

Dorsiflexion range of motion restrictions have been identified as a significant impairment associated with plantar heel pain.[41] One study reported a 5 degree or more dorsiflexion restriction in 78% of his patient population with unilateral plantar fasciitis.[74] Numerous studies have shown that heel cord stretching is one of the most effective treatments for resolving plantar heel pain.[8,11-13,58,60] Plantar fascia-specific stretches have been shown to be even more effective than calf stretches in alleviating plantar heel pain.[75,76] Due to the viscoelastic properties of muscle-tendon units, the duration of the stretch, active warm-up, and the concept of reciprocal inhibition can influence the outcome of stretching.[78,79] Dorsiflexor and plantarflexor muscle weakness via isokinetic testing has also been identified as impairments in chronic plantar fasciitis.[37,77]

Collagen production is probably the key cellular phenomenon that determines recovery from tendinosis.[35] Animal experiments have revealed that loading the tissue improves collagen alignment and stimulates cross-linkage formation, both of which improve tensile strength.[35] Interventions such as friction massage[80-84] and eccentric exercise[34,35,93-95] have been shown to stimulate collagen production and, thus, help to reverse the tendinosis cycle. Therapeutic ultrasound[85-92] has been shown to stimulate angiogenesis in acute wounds yet its effect on chronic tendinopathy has been inconclusive.

Wow! You did it! You made it through an exhaustive review of the literature. As you can see, there should be a good reason why or why not your physical therapist chooses a therapeutic intervention. Congratulations! You are several steps closer to understanding your foot pain.

Please refer to the appendix for a complete list of references

IS IT REALLY INFLAMMATION?

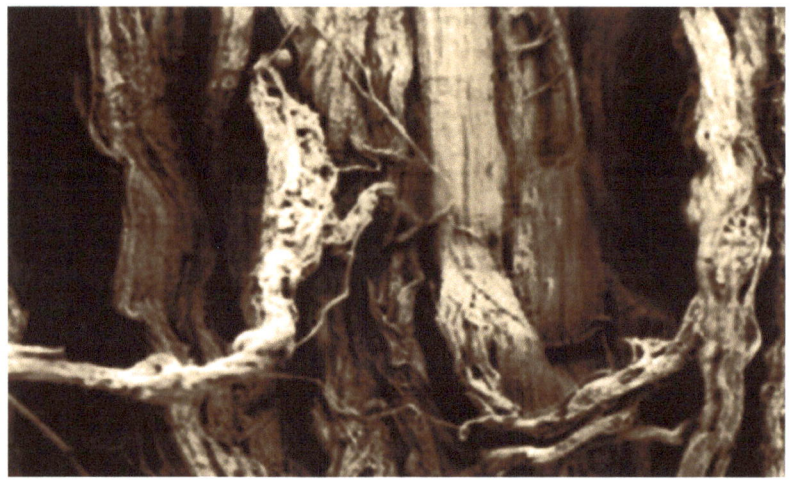

This is a picture of scar tissue.

All physical therapy is NOT created equal. As a physical therapist with over 2 decades of hands-on care, I have tried many approaches in treating soft tissue dysfunction. Tissue stress can be identified objectively through a comprehensive biomechanical evaluation and well as subjectively through a thorough interview with the patient. Patient compliance and therapist experience is paramount in achieving maximum results in minimum time. I strongly feel that the "missing link" in achieving permanent, maximum results is inadequate treatment of soft tissue fibrosis i.e. scar tissue throughout the kinetic chain. Let me explain!

One of the most contentious debates that I have had with physicians as well as physical therapists is the inflammation versus fibrosis debate. Many health care practitioners feel that inflammation is the main source of pain in chronic conditions (greater than 3 weeks). This is evidenced through their long-term use of anti-inflammatory meds, cortisone shots, and the over-use of anti-inflammatory modalities in physical therapy such as iontophoresis and phonophoresis. My main adage as a physical therapist is "there better be a good reason for everything you do!" Evidence-based or research-based treatment is fundamental to our professional growth. I feel that using anti-inflammatory procedures is a very effective strategy in the short-term. It is true that we are our own worst enemies during our hectic lives. Intermittent, acute inflammation can certainly occur. However, what underlying dysfunction is present that predisposes us to this chronic, intermittent pain? What does the research tell us?

Karim Khan,MD in "Time to abandon the "tendonitis" myth", BMJ, 2002, 324(7338):626-7 reports that *"animal studies conclusively demonstrate that, within 2-3 weeks of insult to tendon tissue, inflammatory cells are not present."*

Karim Khan,MD in "Histopathology of common tendinopathies", SportsMed 1999;27(6):393-408 states that *"We conclude that effective treatment of athletes with tendinopathies must target the most common underlying histopathology, TENDINOSIS, a non-inflammatory condition."*

Harvey Lemont,DPM in "Plantar fasciitis", JAPMA 2003;93(3):234-237 states that, after analyzing tissue samples from 50 plantar fascia surgeries, *"Histologic findings are presented to support the thesis that "plantar fasciitis" is a degenerative fasciosis WITHOUT inflammation, not a fasciitis."*

So why are you still taking your anti-inflammatories if you don't have inflammation?

DO YOU REALLY NEED THAT CORTISONE SHOT?

Because no inflammatory cells have been demonstrated in biopsies from chronic tendinopathy, some authors have abandoned the tendonitis "myth" as well as the use of steroids. Recent studies, however, have begun to question this new opinion. The question is NOT whether inflammatory cells exist in chronic tendinopathy. That has been resolved-there is NOT inflammation. The new question is whether cortisone can positively alter the abnormal physiology of scar tissue. Recent placebo controlled, randomized studies of ultrasound-guided peritendinous steroid injections have been shown to be very effective in reducing the pain and thickness of Achilles and patellar tendons in athletes with chronic tendinopathy.

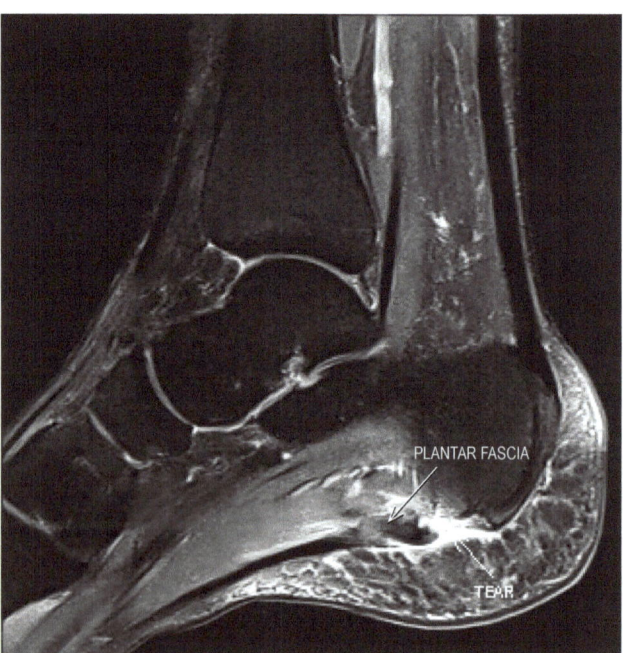

This MRI shows plantar fasciosis. The author notes that although we use the terminology plantar fasciitis, the condition is not inflammatory but is actually a well-documented degenerative condition.

Fredberg et al in "Ultrasonography as a tool for diagnosis, guidance of local steroid injection..", Scand J Rheumatol 2004; 33: 94-101 state that steroid injections "significantly reduced the average diameter of the affected tendons" and "in several cases the thickening of the tendon regresses completely."

Koenig, et al in "Preliminary results of colour Doppler-guided intratendinous glucocorticoid injections..", Scand J Med Sci Sports 2004: 14: 100-106 found that "neovascularization disappears" after ultrasound-guided, intratendinous injections.

The significance of these last two research projects is that steroids have the ability to "shrink" pathological tissue. An interesting question is "should your doctor continue to inject **"blindly"** or use ultrasonography to guide the precise placement of steroid?" Would your results be better and more consistent using ultrasonography?

The "shrinking" of pathological tissue has been associated with a decrease in pain, but it does not stimulate tissue regeneration and strengthening of the pathological tissue. As a result, the patient is susceptible to chronic reinjury. Fredberg states that steroids "*cannot repair degenerative changes*" and attempted to explain "*the high frequency of relapse*" 6 months after the first injection. He now recommends 3-6 months of rehabilitation after injection. In our clinic, the functional regeneration of tissue is our goal! So how does the therapist stimulate tissue regeneration?

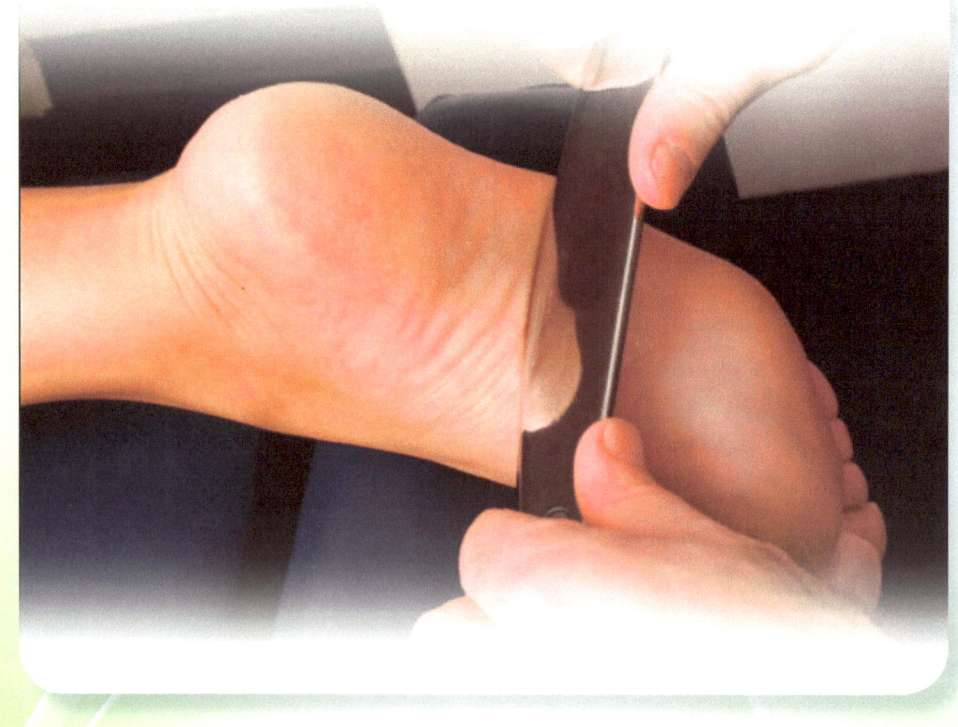

THE EFFECTS OF GRASTON TECHNIQUE

The first step in the process is to identify tissue texture abnormalities. Microscopically, healthy tissue is smooth, longitudinal, and symmetrical in presentation. Scar tissue i.e. fibrosis is laid down by our bodies in a very haphazard and erratic fashion. During palpation, both the clinician and the patient can detect areas of grittiness, nodules, and "knots". A partial tear in the Achilles tendon is thicker, harder, and gritty compared to the healthy side. Fibrosis in the plantar fascia can be felt and heard as you stroke a Graston tool along the central band of the fascia. Once a lesion is detected, I utilize patented and proven techniques such as the *Graston Technique* and *Active Release Technique* to "break up" cross-links, adhesions, and/or restrictions in the tissue. You can view videos of these techniques on my blog at www.orthowellpt.com.

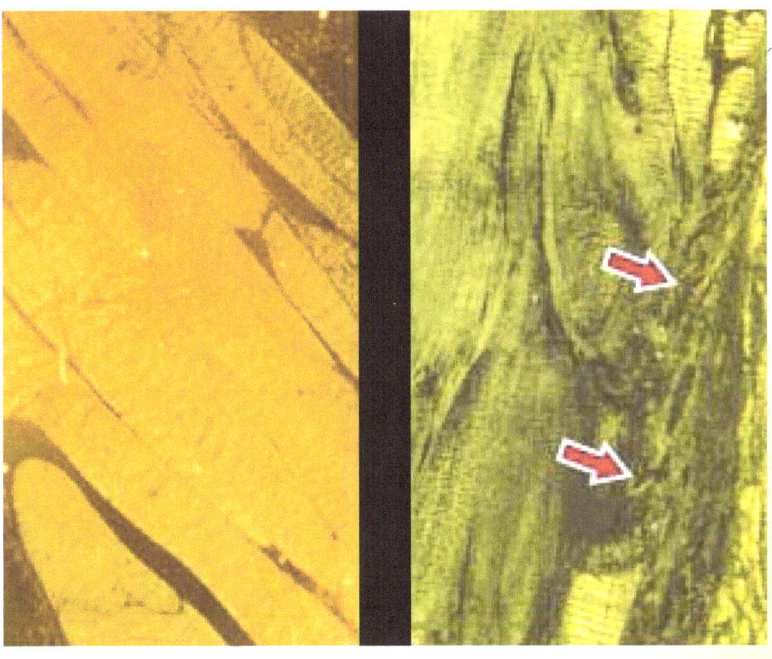

Normal Tendon   Abnormal Tendon

So how does *Graston Technique* work? The instruments are used as an alternative to the therapists fingers to provide deep friction massage. The acoustic properties of the instruments can aide in the diagnostic locating of scar tissue. The deep friction massage of the tools reintroduces microtrauma to the damaged site and sets in motion the healing cascade. During the reactive inflammatory stage, scar tissue can be reabsorbed by the body. In the fibroblastic phase of healing, the damaged tissue is replaced by new collagen and is reformatted through proper stretching and exercise. This "process" can take 3-6 months in chronic cases. Keep in mind that inflammation can occur without healing, but healing of fibrotic tissue cannot occur without inflammation. Deep friction massage initiates the inflammatory cascade to "jump start" the healing process. It has been hypothesized to stimulate the proliferation and activation of fibroblasts. Fibroblasts play a key role in tissue healing because they are responsible for producing the key structural fiber in healthy connective tissue – collagen. So what does the research tell us about the effects of *Graston Technique?*

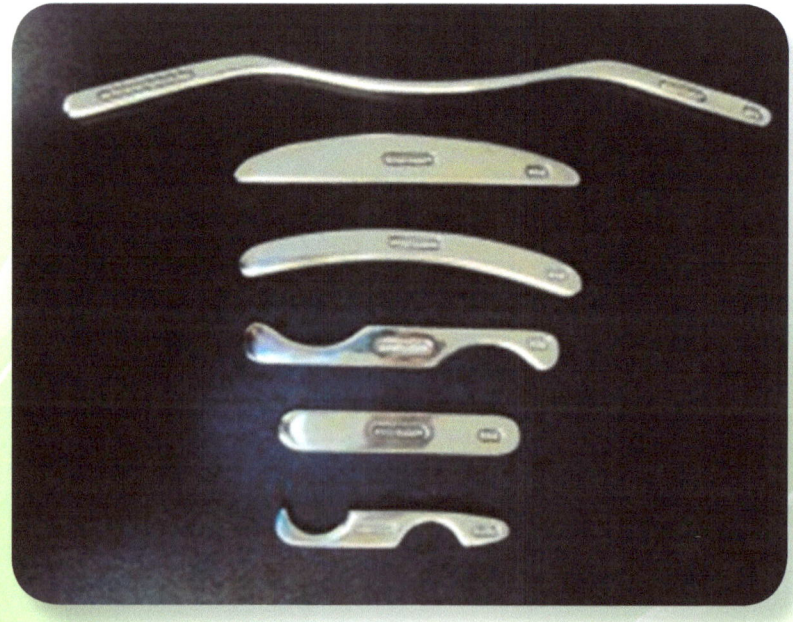

Craig Davidson et al in *"Morphologic and functional changes in rat Achilles tendon following collagenase and GASTM", J Am College Sports Med, 1995;27* showed increased fibroblast proliferation in the Graston group and stated that *"the study suggests that Graston may promote healing via increased fibroblast recruitment."*

Gale Gehlsen et al in *"Fibroblasts responses to variation in soft tissue mobilization pressure", Med Sci Sports Exer, 1999;31:531-535* showed morphological evidence indicating that *"the application of heavy pressure during Graston promoted more fibroblastic proliferation compared to light or moderate pressure."*

Loghmani MT, Warden SJ. Instrument-assisted cross-fiber massage accelerates knee ligament healing. Journal of Orthopaedic & Sports Physical Therapy (JOSPT). 2009 Jul;39(7):506-514. revealed that *"ligaments treated with Graston were found to be 31% stronger and 34% stiffer than untreated ligaments."*

As a result of over 2 decades of asking questions and critically appraising my successes and failures, I have become convinced that the "missing link" in the treatment of chronic pain is the release of scar tissue adhesions. In conjunction with *Graston Technique* and *Active Release Technique*, rehabilitation is accomplished through the functional integration of strengthening, stretching, joint mobilization, cardiovascular exercise, and compliance with a home exercise program. Correcting biomechanical deficiencies with foot orthotics is also a consideration. Most physical therapists do an adequate job of treating pain. Acute pain usually resolves with the most innocuous of therapy interventions. However, the only way to prevent reoccurrence of symptoms is to ensure that every aspect of the dysfunction is being treated in the most comprehensive manner.

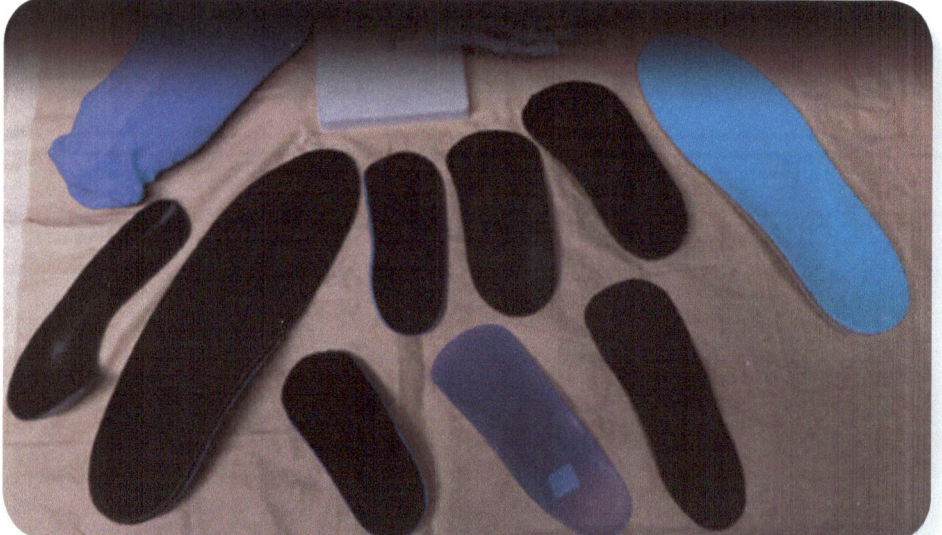

FOOT ORTHOTICS-SHOULD I OR SHOULDN'T I?

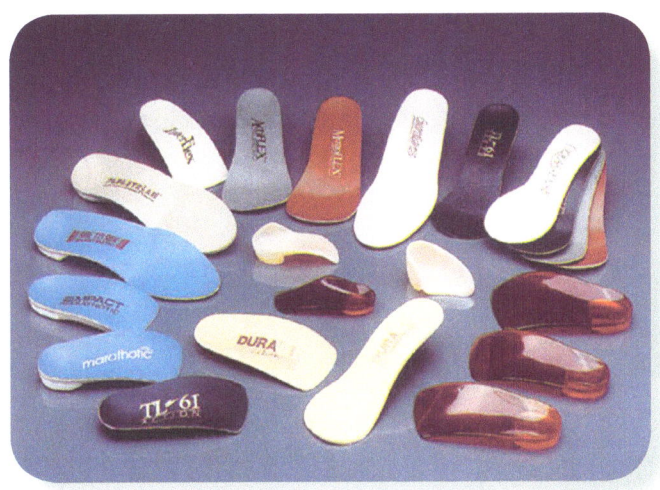

We fabricate a lot of foot orthotics for plantar fasciitis in my physical therapy clinic. There is a very good reason for all that I do in physical therapy as well as with the fabrication of custom foot orthotics for plantar fasciitis. I fabricate custom foot orthotics based on sound biomechanical principles and evidence-based research. Patients are always asking me "so how will foot orthotics help my plantar fasciitis?" Here is the answer! I have included both a clinical description as well as a more basic description in the video on my blog at www.orthowellpt.com. I have included references for several articles that have had a profound influence on my treatment and fabrication philosophy regarding plantar fasciitis. I would like to share my insights with you.

It has been my experience that positive results can be achieved much more quickly for cases of plantar fasciitis using the combination of softer materials to cushion the foot in combination with stiffer, denser materials to redistribute pressures on the foot. My direct molding techniques produce a total contact orthotic which reduces weight bearing pressure on both the heel and forefoot. These findings for total contact orthoses have been confirmed by both *Mueller et al*[10,11] and *Ki et al*[12]. As you can see from my samples on the video, I utilize softer materials as a top layer with the addition of a heel pad on the bottom. I reinforce the arch in order to redistribute pressures up against the talonavicular joint (or midfoot). I utilize a forefoot valgus post (higher on the outside of the forefoot) with a slight reverse Morton extension (ledge under toes 2-5) in order to plantar flex the first ray (big toe lower than the other four toes) and unload both the fascia and 1st MTP joint (big toe joint) As I tell my patients, the foot orthotic is only as good as the shoe you put around it. Our best results with the over-pronating foot are achieved via the combination of motion control shoes and custom orthoses.

In regards to pre-fabricated or over-the-counter foot orthotics, there is some research that has shown pre-fabs to be as effective as custom orthotics in terms of pain reduction. So I tell my patients to start with the pre-fabs first and see what happens. The research is inconclusive regarding the effect of foot orthotics on the motion (kinematics) and the forces (kinetics) that act upon the foot. Lets go into a little more detail.

Research done by *Kogler*[1,2,3] *et al* has been instrumental in determining the appropriate type of rearfoot and/or forefoot posting for foot orthotics for plantar fasciitis. Kogler showed that rearfoot posting(angle in the heel) had little effect on plantar fascia strain, forefoot varus (highest angle under the big toe) posting increased the stress, and forefoot valgus(highest angle under the little toe) posting actually decreased the strain. Kogler concluded that foot orthotics which raised the talonavicular joint(the midfoot) and prevented dorsiflexion of the first ray were most effective in reducing the strain on the central band of the plantar fascia. I recently made orthotics for a patient who said her doctor issued bilateral heel lifts "to take the stress off of the fascia". Kogler actually showed no change in plantar fascia strain using heel lifts. However, heel lifts have been shown by *Trepman et al*[4] in 2000 to decrease the compressive forces in the tarsal tunnel(inside of the ankle). Benno Nigg[5], a researcher in Canada, has also published over 200 articles on biomechanics. He has stated that based on his results, custom foot orthotics, on average, control only 2-3 degrees of motion. This would be his kinematic results, however, he has done a lot of enlightening research on the kinetic effects of foot orthotics. A little bedtime reading for you!

Paul Scherer[6,7],DPM has published several articles on the effects of custom orthotics on the 1st MTP joint(big toe joint). The concept of maintaining the first ray in a plantar flexed position unloads both the 1st MTP joint as well as the plantar fascia. Howard Dananberg[8],DPM has also written several articles on this topic. Doug Richie[9],DPM has been a great resource for the evidence behind the treatment of plantar fasciitis. Dr Richie states that the "most effective foot orthotic for plantar fasciitis is one that hugs against the navicular and flares away from (or plantar flexes) the first ray."

Please refer to the appendix for a complete list of references

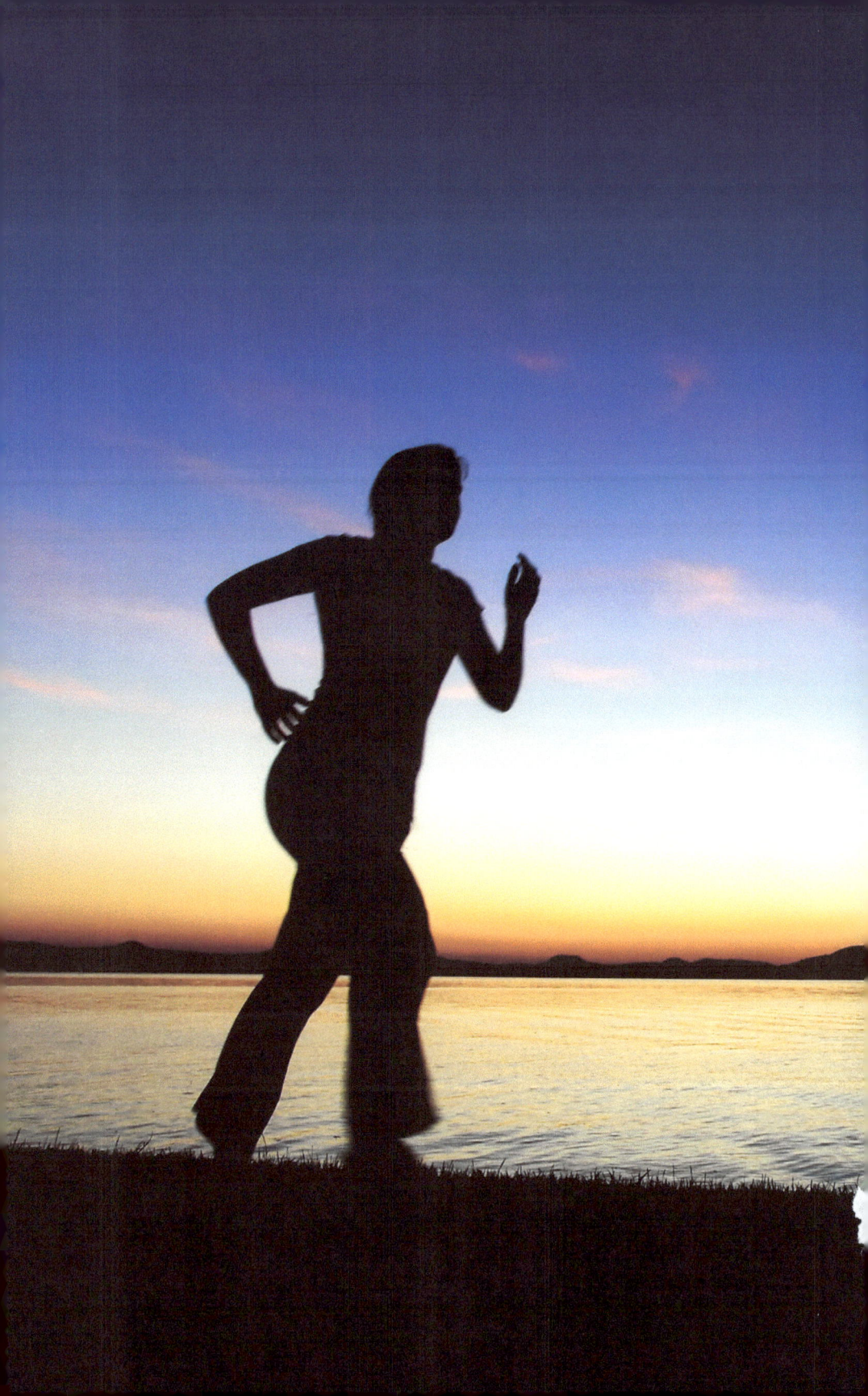

IN CONCLUSION

WOW! You did it! That was a lot of information on the science and evidence behind the treatment of heel pain. Now you are wicked smart! Education is power! You need to understand that there is no definitive treatment for plantar fasciitis nor a panacea in terms of foot orthotics. Over 22 years of treating patients with heel pain, I have been convinced that the therapist needs to take a multi-faceted approach. As was stated at the beginning of this book, *" it is reasonably certain that a condition which has so many different theories of etiology and treatment does not have valid proof of any one cause".* For this reason, I have developed a protocol that works! A protocol that provides a comprehensive approach to the SELF-treatment of plantar fasciitis.

A do-it-yourself plan that will empower you and Cure Yourself Now of Foot Pain!

Check out my website at www.orthowellpt.com or

www.cureyourselfnow-footpain.com to get your plan.

You don't want to wait.

Get started NOW!

THE PLAN

So why do you need a plan? As I explained, you need a plan to resolve your plantar fasciitis once and for all! You need a plan that will prevent reoccurrence of your pain. You need a plan that is multi-faceted and addresses ALL the underlying issues associated with plantar fasciitis.

So what do you get? I have created a self-help DVD because I want to be your coach. I want to take you by the hand and show you step-by-step how YOU can help YOURSELF! Your DVD will include the following:

- Educational videos explaining:
  - HOW and WHY you develop plantar fasciitis
  - HOW foot orthotics work and WHY you may or may not need them
  - HOW the Kinetic Chain works and WHY this is so important
  - HOW to manage your pain and WHY it accelerates your recovery
- Instructional videos explaining your home program which includes:
  - The Trilogy-3 things you will do twice per day
  - The best plantar fascia stretch
  - Self massage and self mobilization of your stiff tissue
  - The best leg muscle stretches
  - Conditioning exercises for your injured tissue
  - Strengthening exercises to prevent return of pain

The only reason that you continue to have pain in your foot is that you have NOT taken action. I have done all the research for you. My clinical expertise is here to guide you.

Your plan of action is only a few clicks away.

Go to www.cureyourselfnow-footpain.com

and order your DVD today!!

APPENDIX

References chapter THE EVIDENCE

1. Riddle DL, Shappert SM: *Volume of ambulatory care visits and patterns of care for patients diagnosed with plantar fasciitis: a national study of medical doctors.* Foot ankle INT 2004, 25(5): 303-310.

2. Dunn Je, Link CL at al: *Prevalence of foot and ankle conditions in a multiethnic community sample of older adults.* Am J Epidem 2004, 159(5):491-498.

3. Badlissi F, Dunn JE et al: *Foot musculoskeletal disorders, pain, and pain-related functional limitations in older persons.* J Am Geriat Soc2005, 53(6):1029-1033.

4. Buchbinder R: *Plantar fasciitis.* NEJM 2004, 350(21):2159-2166.

5. Clement DB et al: *A survey of over-use running injuries.* Phys Sportsmed 1981, 9(5):47-58.

6. Agosta J et al: *Epidemiology of a podiatric sports medicine clinic.* Aust Podiatrist 1994,28(4):93-96.

7. Radford JA, Landorf KB: *Effectiveness of calf muscle stretching for the short-term treatment of plantar heel pain: a randomized trial.* BMC MusculoSkel Dis 2007. 8:36

8. Wolgin M, Cook C: *Conservative treatment of treatment of plantar heel pain: long-term follow-up. Foot & Ankle 1994, 15(3): 97-102.*

9. Martin RL et al: *Outcome study of subjects with insertional plantar fasciitis.* Foot & Ankle 1998, 19(12):803-811.

10. Crawford F, Thomson C: *Interventions for treating plantar heel pain.* Cochrane database of systematic reviews 2007.

11. Gill L: *Plantar fasciitis: diagnosis and conservative management.* J Am Acad Orth Surg 1997, 5(2): 109-117.

12. Gill L et al: *Outcome of nonsurgical treatment for plantar fasciitis.* Foot and ankle international 1996, 17(9):527-532.

13. Davis PF et al: *Heel pain syndrome: results of nonoperative treatment.* Foot and ankle international 1994, 15(10): 531-535.

14. Lynch DM, Goforth WP: *Conservative treatment of plantar fasciitis A prospective study.* JAPMA 1998, 88(8): 375-380.

15. Lapidus, PW, Guidotti FP: *Painful heel: report of 323 patients with 364 painful heels.* Clin Orthop 1965, 39:178-186.

16. Snook GA, Chrisman OD: *The management of sub calcaneal pain.* Clin Orthop 1972, 82:163-168.

17. Atkins D: *A systematic review of treatments for the painful heel.* Rheumatolgy (Oxford) 1999, 38(10): 968-973.

18. Barrett SL: *Should you change your approach to plantar fasciosis.* Podiatry today November 2006.

19. Shapiro SL: *Heel pain management starts with correct differential diagnosis.* Biomechanics September 1997.

20. Meyer J et al: *Differential diagnosis and treatment of sub calcaneal heel pain: a case report.* JOSPT 2001, 32(3): 114-121.

21. Aldridge T: *Diagnosing heel pain in adults.* Am Fam Physician 2004, 70(2): 332-338.

22. Perelman GK et al: *The medial instep plantar fasciotomy.* J Foot Ank Surg 1995, 34(5), 447-510.

23. Richie D: *Offloading the plantar fascia: what you should know.* Podiatry today November 2005.

24. Grasel RP, Schweitzer ME, Kovalovich AM, et al: *MR imaging of plantar fasciitis: edema, tears, and occult marrow abnormalities correlated with outcome.* Am J Roentgenol 173:699, 1999.

25. Scherer PR: Heel spur syndrome. *Pathomechanics and nonsurgical treatment.* J Am Pod Med Assoc 81:68-72, 1991.

26. Schepsis AA, Leach RE, Gorzyca J: *Plantar fasciitis. Etiology, treatment, surgical results, review of the literature.* Clin Orthop 266:185-196, 1991.

27. Almekinders LC and Temple JD. *Etiology, diagnosis, and treatment of tendonitis: an analysis of the literature.* Med Sci Sports Exerc, 1998. 30(8):1183-90.

28. Almekinders LC, Vellema JH, Weinhold PS. *Strain patterns in the patellar tendon and the implications for patellar tendinopathy.* Knee Surg Sports Traumatol Arthrosc, 2002. 10(1):2-5.

29. Puddu G, Ippolito E, Postacchini F: *A classification of Achilles tendon disease.* Am J Sports Med 4:145-150, 1976.

30. Huijbregts PA: *Tendon injury a review.* Jour Man & Manip Ther,Vol 7(2): 71-80, 1999.

31. Khan KM and Maffulli N. *Tendinopathy: an Achilles' heel for athletes and clinicians.* Clin J Sport Med, 1998. 8(3):151-4.

32. Khan KM, et. al. *Time to abandon the "tendinitis" myth.* BMJ, 2002. 324(7338):626-7.

33. Khan KM, Cook JL: *Overuse tendinosis, Not tendinitis. Part 1. A New Paradigm for a difficult clinical problem.* THE PHYSICIAN AND SPORTSMEDICINE - VOL 28 - NO. 5 - MAY 2000.

34. Khan KM, Cook JL, Kiss ZS, et al.: *Patellar tendon ultrasonography and jumper's knee in elite female basketball players: a longitudinal study.* Clin J Sports Med 7:199-206, 1997.

35. Khan KM, Cook JL: *Overuse tendinosis, Not tendinitis. Part 2. Applying the new approach to patellar tendinopathy.* THE PHYSICIAN AND SPORTSMEDICINE - VOL 28 - NO. 6 – June 2000.

36. Lemont H, Ammirati KM, and Usen N. *Plantar fasciitis: a degenerative process (fasciosis) without inflammation.* J Am Podiatr Med Assoc, 2003. 93(3):234-7.

37. Chandler TJ, Kibler WB. A biomechanical approach tothe prevention, treatment and rehabilitation of plantar fasciitis. *Sports Med.* 1999;15:344-352.

38. McPoil TG, Hunt GC. *Evaluation and management of foot and ankle disorders: present problems and future directions.) Orthop Sports Phys Ther.* 1995;21:381-388.

39. Cornwall MC, McPoil TG: *Planter fasciitis: etiology in treatment.* JOSPT, Vol 29(12):756-760, 1999

40. Ross M: *Use of the tissue stress model as a paradigm for developing an examination and management plan for a patient with plantar fasciitis.* JAPMA Vol 92(9):499-506,2002.

41. Young B, Walker M, Strunce J, Boyles R. *A Combined Treatment Approach Emphasizing Impairment-Based Manual Physical Therapy for Plantar Heel Pain:A Case Series.* The Journal of Orthopaedic & Sports Physical Therapy 2004,34(11):725-33.

42. Anderson CR, Morris RL: *Effects of iontophoresis current magnitude and duration on dexamethasone deposition and localized drug retention.* Phys Ther 2003;83:161-170.

43. Costello CT: *Iontophoresis: Applications in transdermal medication delivery.* Phys Ther 1995, Vol 75(6):554-563.

44. Li LC, Scudds RA: *Iontophoresis: an overview of the mechanisms and clinical application.* American College of Rheumatology, 1995, Vol 8(1):51-61.

45. Gudeman SC: *Treatment of planter fasciitis by iontophoresis of 0.4% dexamethasone.* Amer J Sports Med, 1997, Vol 25(3): 312-316.

46. Fredberg U, Bolvig L: *Ultrasonography as a tool for diagnosis, guidance of local steroid injection and, together with pressure algometry, monitoring of the treatment of athletes with chronic jumpers knee and Achilles tendinitis: a randomized, double-blind, placebo controlled study.* Scand J Rheumatol 2004:33;94-101.

47. Acevedo JI, Beskin JL. *Complications of plantar fascia rupture associated with corticosteroid injection. Foot Ankle Int.* 1998;19:91–7.

48. Fredberg U: *Local corticosteroid injection in sport: review of literature and guidelines for treatment.* Scand L Med Sci Sports 1997:7:131-139.

49. Landorf K, Radford J, Keenan A, Redmond A. *Effectiveness of Low-Dye Taping for the Short-term Management of Plantar Fasciitis.* Journal of the American Podiatric Association 2005; 95(6):525-30.

50. Radford J, Burns J, Buchbinder R, Landorf K, Cook C. *The Effect of Low-Dye Taping on Kinematic, Kinetic, and Electromyographic Variables.* Journal of Orthopaedic & Sports Physical Therapy 2006; 36(4):232-41.

51. Lange B: *The effects of low-dye taking on plantar pressures during gait in subjects with navicular drop exceeding 10 mm.* J Orthop Sports Phys Ther • Volume 34 • Number 4 • April 2004.

52. Keenan AM, Tanner CM. *The effect of high-Dye and low-Dye taping on rearfoot motion. J Am Podiatr Med Assoc.* 2001;91:255-261.

53. Vicenzino B, Feilding J, Howard R, Moore R, Smith S. *An investigation of the anti-pronation effect of two taping methods after application and exercise. Gait Posture.* 1997;5:1-5.

54. Vicenzino B, Griffiths SR, Griffiths LA, Hadley A. *Effect of antipronation tape and temporary orthotic on vertical navicular height before and after exercise. J Orthop Sports Phys Ther.* 2000;30:333-339.

55. Gross MT, Byers JM, Krafft JL, Lackey EJ, Melton KM: Impact of custom semi-rigid foot orthotics on pain and disability for individuals with plantar fasciitis. *J Orthop Sports Phys Ther.* 2002;32(4):149-157.

56. Kogler, G. F.; Solomonidis, S. E.; and Paul, J. P.: *Biomechanics of longitudinal arch support mechanisms in foot orthoses and their effect on plantar aponeurosis strain. Clin. Biomech.,* 11: 243-252, 1996.

57. Kogler GF, Veer FB, Solomonidis SE, et al. *The influence of medial and lateral placement of wedges on loading the plantar aponeurosis, An in vitro study*. J Bone and Joint Surg Am. 81:1403-1413, 1999

58. Richie,D. *Offloading the plantar fascia: What you should know*. Podiatry Today, Vol 18. Issue 11, Nov 2005.

59. Landorf KB, Keenan AM: *Effectiveness of foot orthoses to treat chronic fasciitis A randomized trial*. Arch Intern Med 2006, 166(12):1305-10.

60. Pfeffer G: *Comparison of custom and prefabricated orthoses in the initial treatment of proximal plantar fasciitis*. Foot & Ankle Intl Vol 20(4),1999: 214-219.

61. McClay-David I. *Comparison of rearfoot control of custom vs semi-custom foot orthotics*, presented at the International Conference on Foot Biomechanics and Orthotic Therapy. Las Vegas, Nevada Dec 1-3, 2003.

62. Mundermann A, Nigg BM: *Foot orthotics affect lower extremity kinematics and kinetics during running. Clin Biomech*, 2003 Mar;18(3):254-62.

63. DiFabio RP: *Efficacy of manual therapy*. Phys Ther Vol 72(12), 1992: 853-864.

64. Maitland GD: Peripheral manipulation. 2nd Ed Boston ,MA, 1977.

65. Cyriax JH: *Textbook of orthopedic medicine, volume 2: treatment of manipulation, massage, and injection*. Baltimore,MD, 1971.

66. Kaltenborn FM: *Mobilization of the spinal column*. Wellington, New Zealand. 1970.

67. McKenzie R: *The lumbar spine: mechanical diagnosis and therapy*. Spinal publications 1981.

68. Grieve GP: *Mobilization of the spine*, Scotland, 1979.

69. Nield S: *The effect of manipulation on range of movement at the ankle joint*.Scand J Rehab Med 25:161-166, 1993.

70. Pellow JE: *The efficacy of adjusting the ankle in the treatment of subacute and chronic grade one in grade 2 ankle inversion sprains.* J Manip and Physio Ther Vol 24(1): 2001, 17-24.

71. Denegar CR: *The effect of lateral ankle sprain on dorsiflexion range of motion, posterior Talar glide, and joint laxity.* JOSPT Vol 32(4): 166-172, 2002.

72. Soavi R: *The mobility of the proximal tibial – fibular joint.A Roentgen Stereophotogrammeric analysis on six cadaver specimens.* Foot & Ankle Intl Vol 21(4):336-342, 2000.

73. Dananberg H: *Manipulation method for the treatment of ankle equinus.* JAPMA Vol 90(8):385-389, 2000.

74. Amis J: *Painful heel syndrome: radiographic and treatment assessment.* Foot Ankle, 1988, Vol 9(2): 91-95.

75. DiGiovanni BF, Nawoczenski D, Lintal M, Moore E,Murray J, Wilding G, Baumhauer J. *Tissue-SpecificPlantar Fascia-Stretching Exercise Enhances Outcomes in Patients with Chronic Heel Pain: A Prospective, Randomized Study.* The Journal of Bone & Joint Surgery 2003; 85-A(7):1270-77.

76. DiGiovanni BF: *Plantar fascia-specific stretching exercise improves outcomes in patients with chronic plantar fasciitis. A prospective clinical trial with two-year follow-up.* J Bone Joint Surg Am 2006 Aug;88(8):1775-81.

77. Kibler WB: *Functional biomechanical deficits and running athletes with planter fasciitis.* Amer J Sports Med, Vol 19(1): 66-71, 1991.

78. Shrier I, Gossal K: *Myths and truths about stretching.* THE PHYSICIAN AND SPORTSMEDICINE - VOL 28 - NO. 8 - AUGUST 2000.

79. Wiktorsson-Moller M: Effects of warming up, massage, and stretching on range of motion and muscle strength in the lower extremity. Amer J Sports Med, Vol 11(4): 249-252, 1983.

80. Loghmani MT, Warden SJ. *Instrument-assisted cross-fiber massage accelerates knee ligament healing.* Journal of Orthopaedic & Sports Physical Therapy (JOSPT). 2009 Jul;39(7):506-514.

81. Loghmani MT, Kiesel J, Lassiter J, Taylor L, Beaman M, Grogg J, Streeter H, Warden SJ. *Long-term effects of instrument-assisted cross-fiber massage on healing medial collateral ligaments.* JOSPT. 2007 Jan;37(1): A18.

82. Gehlsen GM, Ganion LR, Helfst R. *Fibroblast response to variation in soft tissue mobilization pressure.* Medicine and Science in Sports and Exercise. 1999 Apr;31(4):531-535.1

83. Davidson CJ, Ganion LR, Gehlsen GM, Verhoestra B, Roepke JE, Sevier TL. *Rat tendon morphologic and functional changes resulting from soft tissue mobilization. Medicine and Science in Sports and Exercise.* 1997 Mar;29(3):313-319.1

84. Chamberlain GJ: *Cyriax's Friction massage: a review.* JOSPT, Vol 4(1):16-22, 1982.

85. Speed CA: Therapeutic ultrasound in soft tissue lesions. Rheumatology 2001;40:1331-1336, 2001.

86. Enwemeka CS: *The effects of therapeutic ultrasound on tendon healing, a biomechanical study.* Am J Phys Med Rehab, Vol 68(6):283-287, 1989.

87. Ramirez A: *The effect of ultrasound on collagen synthesis and fibroblast proliferation in vitro.* J Amer Coll Sports Med, 1997.

88. Young SR, Dyson M: *The effect of therapeutic ultrasound on angiogenesis.* Ultrasound in medicine and biology, volume 6(3):261-269, 1990.

89. Crawford F: *How effective is therapeutic ultrasound in the treatment of heel pain.* Annals of the rheumatic diseases, 1996, 55:265-267.

90. Noble JG: *Therapeutic ultrasound: the effects upon cutaneous bloodflow in humans.* Ultrasound in medicine and biology, vol 13(2) 2007: pages 279 to 285.

91. Cunha A: *The effect of therapeutic ultrasound on repair of the Achilles tendon of the rat.* Ultrasound in medicine and biology, vol 27(12) 2001 pages 1691- 1696.

92. Draper DO: *Rate of temperature increase in human muscle during 1 MHz and 3 MHz continuous ultrasound.* JOSPT, Vol 22(4), 142-150, 1995.

93. Stanish WD: *Eccentric exercise in chronic tendinitis.* Clinical orthopedics and related research. Vol 208: 65-68, 1986.

94. Alfredson H, Pietila T, Jonsson P, et al.: *Heavy-load eccentric calf muscle training for the treatment of chronic Achilles tendinosis.* Am J Sports Med 26:360-366, 1998.

95. Ohberg L: *Eccentric training in patients with chronic Achilles tendonosis: normalized tendon structure and decreased thickness at follow-up.* Br J Sports Med 2004;38:8-11.

References chapter FOOT ORTHOTICS-SHOULD I OR SHOULDN'T I?

1. Kogler, G. F.; Solomonidis, S. E.; and Paul, J. P.: *Biomechanics of longitudinal arch support mechanisms in foot orthoses and their effect on plantar aponeurosis strain. Clin. Biomech.,* 11: 243-252, 1996.

2. Kogler GF, Veer FB, Solomonidis SE, et al. *The influence of medial and lateral placement of wedges on loading the plantar aponeurosis, An in vitro study.* J Bone and Joint Surg Am. 81:1403-1413, 1999

3. Kogler GF, Veer FB, Verhulst SJ, Solomonidis SE, Paul JP. *The effect of heel elevation on strain within the plantar aponeurosis: in vitro study.* Foot Ankle Int. 2001 May;22(5):433-9.

4. Trepman E, Kadel NJ: *Effect of foot and ankle position on tarsal tunnel compartment pressure.* Foot Ankle Int 20(11):721, 2000

5. Nigg, B. *Biomechanics of Sport Shoes.* 2011

6. Scherer PR, Sanders J, Eldredge, DE, et al. *Effect of functional foot orthoses on first metatarsophalangeal joint dorsiflexion in stance and gait.* J Am Podiatr Med Assoc 2006;96(6):474-481.

7. Scherer,P. *Recent Advances in Orthotic Therapy.* 2011

8. Dananberg HJ. Functional hallux limitus and its relationship to gait efficiency. *J Am Podiatr Med Assoc.* 1986; 76(11):648-52

9. Richie,D. *Offloading the plantar fascia: What you should know.* Podiatry Today, Vol 18. Issue 11, Nov 2005.

10. Mueller MJ, Hastings M, Commean PK, et al. *Forefoot structural predictors of plantar pressures during walking in people with diabetes and peripheral neuropathy.* J Biomech 2003;36(7):1009-1017.

11. Mueller MJ, Lott DJ, Hastings MK, et al. *Efficacy and mechanism of orthotic devices to unload metatarsal heads in people with diabetes and a history of plantar ulcers.* Phys Ther 2006;86(6):833-842.

12. Ki SW, Leung AK, Li AN. *Comparison of plantar pressure distribution patterns between foot orthoses provided by the CAD-CAM and foam impression methods.* Prosthet Orthot Int 2008;32(3):356-362.

www.ingramcontent.com/pod-product-compliance
Lightning Source LLC
Chambersburg PA
CBHW050850290526
45792CB00002B/597